Living In The Post Antibiotic Era

What Will We Do Now To Survive?

D.W. Graeme

Copyright 2018 by D.W. Graeme
All rights Reserved. No part of this book may be reproduced in any form without permission in writing from the author. Reviewers may quote brief passages in reviews.

The following Book is reproduced below with the goal of providing information that is as accurate and reliable as possible. Regardless, purchasing this Book can be seen as consent to the fact that both the publisher and the author of this book are in no way experts on the topics discussed within and that any recommendations or suggestions that are made herein are for entertainment purposes only.

Professionals should be consulted as needed prior to undertaking any of the action endorsed herein.

This declaration is deemed fair and valid by both the American Bar Association and the Committee of Publishers Association and is legally binding throughout the United States.

Furthermore, the transmission, duplication or reproduction of any of the following work including specific information will be considered an illegal act irrespective of if it is done electronically or in print.

This extends to creating a secondary or tertiary copy of the work or a recorded copy and is only allowed with express written consent from the Publisher. All additional right reserved.

The information in the following pages is broadly considered to be a truthful and accurate account of facts and as such any inattention, use or misuse of the information in question by the reader will render any resulting actions solely under their purview. There are no scenarios in which the publisher or the original author of this work can be in any fashion deemed liable for any hardship or damages that may befall them after undertaking information described herein.

Additionally, the information in the following pages is intended only for informational purposes and should thus be thought of as universal. As befitting its nature, it is presented without assurance regarding its prolonged validity or interim quality. Trademarks that are mentioned are done without written consent and can in no way be considered an endorsement from the trademark holder.

Contents

Introduction 7

Chapter 1:
When the "Miracle" Started 9

Chapter 2:
Where is the "Miracle" Now? 19

Chapter 3:
What We Are Fighting
- Level Urgent 30

    HAZARD LEVEL – URGENT
    30

    CLOSTRIDIUM DIFFICILE (Cdiff) 33

    Carbapenem-Resistant Enterobacteriaceae
    (CRE) 40

    CRE Risk Factors 43

    Signs and symptoms of Infections with CRE 43

    Gonorrhea 48

        Chapter 4: What We Are Fighting – Level
        Serious 54

    HAZARD LEVEL – SERIOUS
    54

    Multidrug-Resistant Acinetobacter 56

    Drug-Resistant Campylobacter 58

Fluconazole-Resistant Candida 62

Extended Spectrum Enterobacteriaceae (ESBL)..68

Vancomycin-Resistant Enterococcus (VRE)74

Multidrug-Resistant Pseudomonas aeruginosa..80

Drug-Resistant Non-Typhoidal Salmonella 84

Drug-Resistant Shigella.............................94

Drug-Resistant Streptococcus pneumoniae97

Methicillin-Resistant Staphylococcus Aureus (MRSA)...100

Drug-Resistant Tuberculosis 109

Chapter 5:
Where Do We Go from Here?.....................113

Conclusion 118

Introduction

We are now living in the Post Antibiotic Era. Antibiotic resistance is at all time high. Like it or not, we are now facing what was once termed in a popular hit song, "(On) The Eve of Destruction." Unfortunately, it will be a destruction of our own making.

We have caused it all.

This book is for your education, to arm you with the key information to keep you safe, as to what we are facing at this moment in time. This book will show you what you, as an individual, need to do to protect yourself and your family.

All of the details this book can be backed up by going to the Center for Disease Control Website or the World Health Organization website, and doing your own research there.

It is time we act.

There are no new generation antibiotics headed to the market and to make things worse, we have had any new antibiotics since the 1980s. We are in grave trouble as a World.

It is my hope, that this book will help you make better decisions and keep you safe in the coming years, as we hit the proverbial "Tipping" point of medicine.

Chapter 1: When the "Miracle" Started

Today, so many things are taken for granted, and one of the BIG things that we take for granted is Antibiotics. Of course, there are many things we take for granted as a society, but this one thing alone can be deadly.

If we start to run a fever, we call the doctor and ask for a script for antibiotics, because we are too busy to see the doctor, or we go to the office and tell them just to give us some pills, so we can get back to living.

We take a few of the pills (not all of them) and call the doctor again, angry because we are not already well in two days. We live in an instant world. There is ready-to-eat (fast food), instant pudding, instant coffee, and the list could go on forever that has made us expect to be instantly well. Something is wrong with this "instantness" of society.

We had soldiers that fought for us in WWII that seemed to grow up in another time and another world. These were the same men who would have watched their children die of blood poisoning from a mere splinter and yet, didn't even think about a bullet wound on the battlefield.

It is amazing how those people survived some of the things they did, including diarrhea out on the battlefields and bronchitis along with a host of other infections that befell them. So, to this age group, antibiotics were a drug that was nothing less than a "miracle."

You are going to think it started with penicillin, but it did not. It began with sulfa drugs.

There was a German doctor of pathology who developed sulfa drugs and tested it out on his own family. In 1935, Hildegard, the German doctor's daughter who was six years old, stuck her palm with what you would think of as clean, embroidery needle. It caused a terrible infection that encompassed her entire arm.

The surgeons there kept opening the abscess and draining it, but it did no good. The little girl lay there with lapses in and out of consciousness, and they had started to talk amputation. The father, the German doctor, wanted to try his drug, the sulfa drug he had named Prontosil. In a matter of days, the little girl was able to go home from the hospital all because the drug saved her arm and her life.

Following that event, it was not even a year later, as a matter of fact, that this same drug cured Franklin Delano Roosevelt Jr., who was the son of the then American President of the dreaded strep. He had a severe case, and when he took the sulfa drug, he was cured. The drug became an instant success, and the press in the United States made sure everyone knew about Prontosil.

Prontosil was found to be useful and effective for many conditions from pneumonia to scarlet fever and many more. It had the reputation as many said to "pull folks from the grave."

At the time when the Japanese bombed Pearl Harbor December 7, 1941, it was used in treating the wounded soldiers. They soon allowed all American soldiers that went into combat to carry packets of sulfa powder and pills in their own first- aid kit.

If you have watched any old WWII films, you have probably noticed a soldier opening a packet of something and sprinkling it in his wounds. Now you know what it was that he was doing. No one knows if it did any good out on the battlefield and we will never know, but for that time, it was better than nothing.

The sulfa drug was effective in keeping the outbreaks of diarrhea under control during the Guadalcanal and then just as efficacious during a meningitis outbreak while they were staying at a British Military Base.

During WWI almost 50,000 U.S. soldiers died from pneumonia, influenza, bronchitis and many other diseases that if there had only been the sulfa drug, it would have made a difference.

When WWII came along, and there were two times as many women and men that were in uniforms, there were only 1,265 deaths from those diseases. The only thing that it could be contributed to was sulfa.

However, as we all know, good and great things cannot last. Many of the diseases the sulfa had worked so well on had started becoming resistant. Why, because the sulfa drug was used for EVERYTHING. To keep from getting a sexually transmitted disease, some of the soldiers thought if they would just take a couple of the tablets before they went out for a night on the town that it would take care of that little problem. It caused gonorrhea to become resistant to the sulfa drug.

The next wonder drug to come along was penicillin. Alexander Fleming, a microbiologist, came back from vacation in 1928 and happened to notice on a petri dish he was growing the bacteria Staphylococcus that some mold had started growing on the plate as well and where it had grown there a halo formed where the bacteria had died.

Fleming wrote a paper on this discovery, but it went unnoticed until about 1938 when an Australian pharmacologist and a Jewish refugee took an interest. They worked with Fleming and proved that penicillin was not toxic and could kill a wide variety of bacteria and especially the bacteria that caused gangrene.

No one could figure out how to mass produce the penicillin until it was brought to the United States to the town of Peoria, Illinois where they had an abundance of corn. Corn was used as the primary ingredient to help create the mold needed to make the penicillin.

In the fall of 1943, it was announced that Penicillin appeared to be easy, but the quick cure for syphilis and it was also used for the sulfa resistant gonorrhea.

Sexually transmitted diseases were unchecked during wartime and finding a cure that would take care of the problem raised a question as to how to allocate the supplies of the penicillin. Should it go to the "battlefield or bordellos?"

In discussions during that time, the bordello made the most sense. Churchill, however, ordered that the battlefield would come first.

It was noted that the German soldiers were experiencing the same problems on the same levels with venereal diseases, but they had no efficacious medicine to cure their ills. There are some who theorize that the German troop's strength was what helped the Allied Forces win during the battles in the later part of the war.

Back in the United States on August 11, 1943, doctors were saying that a two-year-old little girl from New York who had blood poisoning would not live seven hours when a newspaperman caught wind of the story. He badgered the guys in Washington to let this little girl have enough of the medicine to try and save her life. Little Patricia recovered in a matter of hours.

It caught the interest of a man by the name of John Smith, who had lost his 16-year-old daughter before the development of Penicillin. So, in September of 1943, Pfizer bought an old ice factory in New York. Eighteen months later this plant was turning out penicillin at the magnitude of 7,000 gallons from each of the fourteen fermenters.

It was four months, on June the sixth of 1944, when the Allied troops stormed the beaches of Normandy carrying penicillin with them.

It sounds crazy to hint that penicillin helped us win WWII, but it is felt that the soldiers had to have felt that way to some degree, especially those who were wounded.

All the military surgeons felt like a miracle had been dropped in their hands when penicillin was delivered to them. When the war first started, and a convoy of wounded would come in, the surgeons would look at the incoming injured, removing dressings and searching for "clean" wounds.

It would have been a terrible decision to make to weed out who was too infected and probably wouldn't make it and turn them away to leave them to die and those they thought they had a shot at saving.

The treatment used if someone had a deep wound would be to drain the wound and leave it open to heal. In wartime, infections were deadly most of the time. If you were lucky and survived, it could take months.

However, things changed when the wounded troops had penicillin out in the battlefield to start receiving, and the surgeons back at the field hospital came to realize that they could wait till the soldier was on the operating table to inspect the wound. Surgeons were awestruck by how good the wounds looked and how much less pain the soldiers seemed to have.

At the field hospitals, it became routine when the soldier went to surgery all that had to be done was clean up the wound, sprinkle it with the penicillin powder, then stitch them up and send the soldier along so he could recover with follow up penicillin injections.

It changed outcomes for the soldiers immensely. Surgeons were operating on 30-40 cases a day; gangrene was now occurring in only 1.5 cases/thousand.

German prisoners, since penicillin at that time was still scarce, was given sulfa and they were suffering from gangrene at the rate of 20-30/thousand.

Chapter 2: Where is the "Miracle" Now?

Sitting back, and watching the faces of an audience being told about antibiotic resistance (and what we are facing), there is a split in audience. Some of the audience understands and believes what is being told to them, and show concern. Others, however, do not believe a word being told to them, and feel that Big Pharma will come out with more drugs... and save the Day.

Many people, do not want to be confronted with the reality of the situation as it faces them. They had rather not know and go on living life as it is and let someone else take care of it.

One type of bacteria can be growing next to another strain of bacteria in someone's body, and can transfer its DNA to the other; therefore, transferring the resistant pattern, they may carry onto another bacteria nearby.

Bacteria may not have a brain so to speak, but they have been present since the dawn of time and will be here long after we are gone. They seem to be able to adapt to any situation and survive.

We are facing a healthcare crisis worldwide as we have never encountered before. The sad part is the there is no one reason for this crisis either. There are a multitude of reasons including:

- Patients are not taking the entire amount of antibiotics prescribed to them by their doctor, so they can save some for their next infection. (This does not make a complete kill of that bacteria and allows what bacteria that was not killed off to become resistant to that antibiotic.)

- Patients taking other family members antibiotics for their infections that may not even be appropriate for the infection that they have. (Making the organism they are infected with resistant to the antibiotic they have just taken.)

- Buying lots of antibiotics on a cruise while they hop off at one of the stops. Everyone does this as antibiotics in other countries do not require a prescription, and they are CHEAP. $5-$10 for a z-pack. They also buy for others while on the cruises. It is easy to understand this as medicines in other countries are cheaper than co-pays on most insurances or they may not be covered under the policy.

- Mothers are demanding antibiotics for their child when the child has a viral infection. Antibiotics are only for treating bacteria. They WILL NOT kill a virus! You might as well drink water. The doctor with all the competition for patients now feel if he does not do what the mother asks will lose them as a patient.

- Antibiotics in cattle, pig, sheep, turkey, and some chicken food. Usually, gentamicin is the antibiotic used. It has a two-fold purpose. To be used as a preservative and to keep the animal healthy and not catch any infections before going to market for slaughter. Which, at the time you eat the product you will be ingesting the antibiotics in the meats as well as all the hormones they are given as well.

- People are buying antibiotics on the black market. They purchase antibiotics from other countries where you do not have to have a prescription. The other countries do not care if they are paid.

- Some people who must have repeat admits to the hospital due to severe health issues and given multiple antibiotics for their illness. Because the patient is subjected to so many different antibiotics, laying in a hospital bed, with their wounds not healing, it begs for more different antibiotics and allows the patient to become a breeding ground for drug-resistant strains of bacteria.

So, there you have it. The short list of reasons. It could go on and on. Each cell of bacteria has 20,000 ways of remaking itself (DNA) to survive, to become resistant. No doubt this mechanism has served the bacteria well since the beginning of time.

If you remember, last year, Playboy founder Hugh Hefner passed away. He was 91 years old. His death certificate lists two causes of death. One was cardiac arrest, and the other was a bacterial infection.

His infection was from E. coli, a bacterium that lives in our gut. Hefner held out for six days with the infection, but the antibiotics would not touch the E. coli, and his death certificate stated the e. coli as "highly resistant."

If you research of E. coli, you will find that most people are exposed to it by contaminated water or food. Your raw vegetables and beef that is undercooked are your two most common routes. The infection usually will last about a week. However, in older people and young children, it can be deadly and start to produce a toxin that will hemolyze organs.

The raw vegetables could become contaminated in a variety of ways. One of them is if they are handled by field hands who have gone to the bathroom facilities and failed to wash their hands before they return to handle the vegetables and then the vegetables are eaten raw, then you will probably have had a good chance of ingesting feces that was on the fresh veggies. Hard to think about is it not?

Public Health of Nevada became involved in a case of a woman who had an infection that the doctors could not cure. The testing revealed that this bacteria superbug was throughout her entire body and could fend off 26 different antibiotics.

It was eventually tested with every antibiotic available within the United States but to no avail. Unfortunately for this patient, she expired.

This patient was infected with CRE – a bacteria called carbapenem-resistant Enterobacteriaceae. It is a bacteria that lives in your colon that for some reason had become resistant to antibiotics that they call carbapenems which are a "last line" of defense when nothing else will work. Doctors call it a "nightmare bacteria."

The hospital worker who has multi-drug resistant TB and will not take his medications and did not notify his employer of this issue until it was found in routine testing. He had been around thousands before it was discovered.

How can someone in their right mind decide to do this to others? I will never understand.

However, all of that aside, the situation has come to such a global threat that the United Nations called a high-level meeting. It is only the fourth time they have called a meeting in regards to a worldwide health issue since the United Nations has been formed.

It is estimated that this uncontrollable 'antibiotic resistance' will "kill more than cancer" does at present; in our coming years. The numbers tell us that 700,000 die every year from antibiotic resistance. This number is anticipated to explode by 2050 to 10 million. What do our children and grandchildren of today have facing them?

The World Health Organization has warned that gonorrhea, a sexually transmitted disease is becoming untreatable due to its resistance to antibiotics.

Most people, the consumer, do not realize that antibiotics cannot be whipped up in the laboratory as needed for each new resistant organism that appears on the horizon.

Antibiotics we use are based on the chemicals we find out in nature, that are produced by other organisms like bacteria in the soil, such as the case of fungi and penicillin.

The organisms have to be identified in nature before they can be synthesized in a laboratory in a test tube and then go through the rigorous ten year testing period set by the FDA.

The sad part it seems, is that when we find a new antibiotic, the organism quickly finds a way to be resistant.

As of this writing, the Miracle we knew during WWII no longer exists. The Miracle has been misused and abused so much that it is no longer of any benefit. To some, they have taken the Miracle drugs so much they have become allergic to the point of anaphylaxis, so the Miracle drug is now a death sentence.

We are on the brink of the cliff where there will be no antibiotics that will work. Having worked with physicians and CDC on cases that no antibiotics were available, that would treat the patient's infection makes it a reality. In those cases, the physician would try to hit the organism in three different directions with three different antibiotics; not knowing if what he was doing was going to work but there was no other choice and something had to be tried to save the patient's life.

Each drug would affect the bacteria differently, and all we could do was cross our fingers and see if this would save the patient. In some cases it did, in others, the attempt just would not work. The bacteria won.

In the chapters to come, you will be introduced to some strains of bacteria that are our enemies right now, in order to educate you so that you may be prepared and not walk "blindly into that good night".

As a prior Infection Control Practitioner, you may think that I am screaming wolf. I promise you, I am not. I have worked many of the cases about to be discussed in this book, and realize some of them will be hard to believe.

There are some who make fun in the way we eat and prepare our foods, but there will not be a chance taken for myself or my family. It is not worth it. Too much has crossed our paths.

Chapter 3: What We Are Fighting - Level Urgent

What we are fighting seems ludicrous as it is organisms that were so easy to kill 50 years ago, but now when someone contracts them, they become life-threatening. How can it be, we ask?

Here, and in the next chapters, is the updated list of CDCs latest organisms that have become our real enemies and what we must do our best to try and avoid:

HAZARD LEVEL – URGENT

- Clostridium Dificile (CDIFF)
- Carbapenem-Resistant Enterobacteriaceae (CRE)

- Neisseria gonorrhoeae

This list was last updated April 14, 2017.

We will embark on the following chapters to identify what CDC considers our riskiest threats to our country and planet.

It can seriously makes one feel that we are facing the antibiotic apocalypse. If this is the case, we have regressed to the dark ages as far as antibiotics and our far technologically advanced countries will not have the means to save patients with infections.

We will soon be hearing from physicians, "We are so very sorry, but we have nothing to use to cure you and your infection. We have done everything we can do. All that we can do now is keep you as comfortable as possible."

If you have never been infected with any of the above-listed organisms, then be ever so thankful for that fact.

CLOSTRIDIUM DIFFICILE (Cdiff)

These bacteria usually affect the older generation, but it has been seen in the very young and healthy that have NO risk factors to have the organism.

There are some who carry the C. diff organism around in their colon, but it never makes them sick. Do not let this fool you however because the carrier can still spread the infection.

If you are going to contract it, you will start to notice the signs in about five-ten days usually after starting an antibiotic. However, do not be surprised if it does not start for two months.

If you get a mild to moderate infection, you will suffer from some mild stomach cramps, and your belly will be tender. Two or three times a day you will have very watery diarrhea.

If the infection is severe, you usually become dehydrated and most of the time must be hospitalized. It causes your colon to become so inflamed that it starts to bleed and to make pus (pseudomembranous colitis).

Some of the signs you will encounter will be:

- Weight loss (some say up to 20 pounds a week or more)
- Loss of appetite
- Dehydration
- Nausea
- Pus or blood in patient's stool
- Fever
- Rapid heart rate
- Stomach cramping, pain (feels like being stabbed by dull knife)
- Abdomen swells due to all the inflammation
- Kidney failure
- White count increases

- The frequency of stools sometimes as often as every 20 minutes.

C. diff can be found all around us in our environment – animal feces, human feces, water, air, soil, food products, and processed meats.

If you have never been around someone with Cdiff, you will never forget the smell. It is atrocious, and you will feel that they most certainly will die. Their diarrhea is explosive, projectile, and frequent. They are in terrible pain from this mean organism. You would swear they have swallowed a pack of razor blades. Alcohol gel will not touch the eradication efforts for Cdiff.

The mechanism of transmission is that the C. diff spores which have a hard-outer shell are released in feces, and from there it gets spread to objects, surfaces, and food when people that are infected do not thoroughly wash their hands.

The spores can live in a room for months. If you happen to touch a light switch for example that has a spore on it and not realizing get the spore in your mouth and swallow it, you can become contaminated.

About the only disinfectant that will penetrate and kill the spores of C. diff is Clorox. If it does not contain sodium hypochlorite, it cannot penetrate the spore to kill the C. diff bacteria. Contact time with Clorox is anywhere from three to ten minutes depending on the product you purchase. I make my own chlorox solution.

Unfortunately, there is a new aggressive strain that releases many more toxins than the other strains do. The new strain seems to be more resistant to some of the medications that are usually given for C. diff and have not had any risk factors. Since its appearance in 2000, it has caused several outbreaks.

C. diff can cause severe dehydration, kidney failure, toxic megacolon, bowel perforation, and even death.

What to do to keep from contracting C. diff? Wash your hands, if you are around someone that has C. diff make sure that all surfaces are decontaminated using chlorine bleach. Avoid taking unnecessary antibiotics if possible. Healthcare workers know what precautions to take.

What happens if you get the drug-resistant strain of the C. diff and there is no antibiotic to be found that will work? Currently, there is Fecal Microbial Transplantation (Bacteriotherapy)

Most patients usually prefer it is a family member. This person should not:

- Have taken any antibiotics for six months
- Be in an immunocompromised position
- Had no body piercing or tattooing for six months
- Never been a drug user
- Never had a high-risk behavior sexually
- Never been in jail
- Have not been traveling to an endemic area lately
- Cannot have IBD or chronic gastrointestinal disorders

Moreover, the donor will have to be screened by their physician for the following:
- Stool Tests: parasites, ova; C. diff PCR; CC&S; antigen for giardia
- Blood Tests: Serology for Hepatitis A, B, C; RPR; HIV

- The donor should know that their insurance may not pay for the testing and they may be asked to pay upfront out of their pocket before the transplant. They will need to check with their insurance company.

If the stool from the donor is considered cleared; there will be a nasoduodenal tube advanced down through the colon. As the tube is being taken out the donor stool is released into the recipient's colon.

There is a new drug called Firvanq which is an oral liquid vancomycin to be taken for C. diff. However, this is not for the resistant strain. How quickly Cdiff will become resistant to this treatment remains to be seen.

Carbapenem-Resistant Enterobacteriaceae (CRE)

CRE is a strain of bacteria which is a member of germs that are common all over the world. They colonize (live in harmony) in the mucosal membranes of animals and human's inclusive of their gastrointestinal tracts and sometimes you will even find it on the skin.

Sadly, CRE contains a unique genetic composition that helps the bacteria to produce the enzyme that will protect CRE germs from one of the most potent antibiotics: carbapenem.

There are other strains of bacteria that can transfer this genetic code to other Enterobacteriaceae: Klebsiella pneumonia, E. coli, and we must also include Pseudomonas aeruginosa making them all carbapenemase resistant.

What doctors have found that is the CRE germs are pretty much like MRSA and could lower the bacteria being susceptible to several antibiotics. It causes us to use several antibiotics to try and treat CRE infections that could cause the patient to develop a C. diff infection on top of what they are already fighting.

This organism is scary because in 2015; it killed two patients and five others were severely infected but survived. It was felt that all these patients were exposed to a contaminated endoscope that had been used in treating pancreatic-biliary diseases.

An endoscope is very hard to clean as it has many small surfaces to get into to grasp every little organism that you cannot see cleaned out. You may think you have it cleaned out, but an organism can be hiding in one of the crevices and then they are put into a machine that will clean them further and hung up to dry, draining all the water out.

CRE is considered dangerous. It is transferred person to person by contact with dirty, contaminated instruments in the hospital, on someone's skin, or with contaminated feces.

Some people do not realize this can be picked up at salad bars if someone that carries this goes to the bathroom and does not wash their hands appropriately before returning to work and then puts food out on the salad bar. The feces can be disposed microscopically on the different items of the salad bar.

It can also be dispersed by people who are eating at the salad bar handling the ladles and picking at food while at the bars.

CRE Risk Factors

- If you have been around someone that is colonized or infected with CRE.
- If you have had a procedure with an endoscope.
- People who have had some type of treatment outside of the U.S.
- People that have taken multiple antibiotics recently, especially in the hospital.
- People who work in healthcare.

Signs and symptoms of Infections with CRE

It all depends on what organ system has been infected with the superbug. If it is in a kidney or kidneys, you will have flank pain and fevers. If you have a wound infection with CRE, there will be pus production and pain.

We must not forget however that these same symptoms can pop up with other types of readily treatable bacterial infections. Being as there are no "specific symptoms of CRE infection" there seem to be problems that might develop that should make a doctor suspect that it might be an infection caused by CRE.

Here are some of them:

- (bloodstream infections) – causing septic shock
- Hypotension (low blood pressure
- (sepsis) life-threatening infection
- High fever
- Severe UTI (urinary tract infection)
- Severe pneumonia
- Cyanosis (skin that is turning blue to gray)
- Finding organisms with this resistance to many antibiotics inclusive of carbapenem.

If someone becomes infected with this organism, a primary care physician can be involved in the process of the treating, but they should be consulting with an infectious disease specialist, a critical care specialist, and a pharmacist at the minimum.

To diagnose a CRE infection, a blood culture must be carried out. The culture will show what bacteria will grow out that is causing the infection. To find out if this organism is resistant to antibiotics a sensitivity test must be run. If the superbug is resistant, there will be growth right up to the drug disc dropped on the petri dish of bacteria you have plated out or in the more sensitive new machinery for biologics in the lab, the tube will be clear.

One of the drugs, of course, will be carbapenem. Sometimes a test called PCR (polymerase chain reaction) may be ordered to identify what type of bacteria is causing this patient's infection.

As far as treating organisms that are resistant to carbapenem-resistant Enterobacteriaceae has become very difficult. Some physicians will pick a group of antibiotics that act like they may have some ability to inhibit or kill this dangerous bacterium from multiplying. For instance, they may try antibiotics like temocillin, Monurol, Tygacil, polymyxins, and some aminoglycosides that have had some success in treating the infection from CRE.

Since we have very few pharma companies that are even trying to develop new antibiotics, we can almost be assured that the bacteria will tip the scales in their favor, and it will not go well for the infected patients who are treated with the same old antibiotics that we have used for a long time.

If CRE is identified early and treated appropriately, the prognosis could be fair, but if CRE has already reached the bloodstream, **death usually occurs 40-50% of the time.**

Gonorrhea

Antibiotic resistance is pushing us even faster to where we will soon have a gonorrhea that cannot be treated. It has already become resistant to our last line of treatment, azithromycin, and cephalosporin.

Some of the countries that are what we call the high-income countries have already seen cases of gonorrhea that they have not been able to treat with all known antibiotics. It is just the tip of The Titanic's iceberg. The reason to discuss this is in the high-income countries we have surveillance and can keep up with the resistance strains whereas the low-income countries have nothing of the sort and gonorrhea is an everyday household word.

The WHO says there are only three possible antibiotics in the pipeline to *maybe* be approved one day to treat gonorrhea, but who knows if it will ever make it out of the pipeline.

Current statistics are that 78 million people are infected with this sexually transmitted disease each year. It is inclusive of 4.5 million-Eastern Mediterranean region, 4.7 million- European region, 11 million- in both Americas, 11.4 - Africa, 11.4 million- Southeast Asia, and 35.2 million- Western Pacific.

While practicing as an Infection Control Nurse Practitioner, there were many young adults coming to me with what was considered serious questions. Some of them being, "can we still contract a sexually transmitted disease if we only have oral sex?" My answer to them was, "YES."

The reason for my answer was that the disease, in this case, would not take up residence where you might expect, but it had the opportunity to take up residence anywhere along the way starting in the mouth where there was a break in the mucous membrane for any sexually transmitted pathogen to enter. It was all too easy to transmit. There is almost always a bleeding gum or sore spot in someone's mouth that the organism can enter and therefore have a direct pathway into your bloodstream leading to septicemia.

Seriously, tell me these numbers are NOT staggering to you? 11 million in the Americas. Let's say there were 5.5 million in the United States of America alone. That would be the equivalent of 110,000 people with gonorrhea per state.

You would think that in a country as educated as the United States that Neisseria gonorrhea would not still be a problem. It is one STD that lets itself be known to male or female easily and therefore nothing that hides as some

STDs, so you are unknowing if you have a sexual partner.

Working with patients who had put off coming to the doctor for so long that when they were sure they had a sexually transmitted disease; when we would put their feet up in stir-ups a large bucket had to be placed under them. The exudate running from them ran out so quickly and copiously that the only thing that could catch and hold it was a large bucket. I do not relay this information to sicken anyone; I relay this, so you can understand the seriousness of what is happening in the real world.

Also, understand that some of the STDs are so serious that they can leave scarring that may lead to problems relating to fertility.

However, let me veer off gonorrhea for just a moment and say that gonorrhea is not the only sexually transmitted disease we see that has become terrible. We are seeing so many different types of organisms being cultured from the genital regions that it is frightening as to what can be transmitted sexually in this day. Organisms that have never before been cultured as sexually transmitted diseases before are now rearing their ugly heads and showing themselves to us.

We are now culturing Salmonella, Shigella and other organisms that reside in the colon and stool from vaginal and penile exudate.

Because of the excessive resistance of gonorrhea, the World Health Organization has recommended for around the world to use a two-antibiotic regime to treat drug-resistant gonorrhea with azithromycin and ceftriaxone.

We cannot stress the use of condoms enough and even at that if there is not very careful handling before and after intercourse the bacteria can quickly be passed.

The three drugs in the pipeline are Solithromycin which is a fluoroketolide taken orally that can kill gonorrhea, Mycoplasma genitalium, and Chlamydia trachomatis.

The second drug is Zoliflodacin is a first-class spiro pyrimidine trione topoisomerase II inhibitor that shows activity against several pathogens. The phase 2 trial showed great promise with a 98-100% cure rate, and more than 90% of the participants in the trial were men.

The third drug is Gepotidacin is a topoisomerase II inhibitor that seems to have a significant effect against several drug-resistant bacteria, and that includes MRSA, ESBL

Enterobacteriaceae, along with gonorrhea.

Chapter 4: What We Are Fighting – Level Serious

HAZARD LEVEL – SERIOUS

- Multidrug-Resistant Acinetobacter
- Drug-Resistant Campylobacter
- Fluconazole-Resistant Candida
- Extended Spectrum Enterobacteriaceae (ESBL)
- Vancomycin-Resistant Enterococcus (VRE)
- Multidrug-Resistant Pseudomonas aeruginosa
- Drug-Resistant Non-Typhoidal Salmonella
- Drug-Resistant Shigella
- Methicillin-Resistant Staphylococcus Aureus (MRSA)
- Drug-Resistant Streptococcus pneumoniae

- Drug-Resistant Tuberculosis

Multidrug-Resistant Acinetobacter

Some species of Acinetobacter usually inhabits human's mucous membranes, soil, and human skin. Some strains can be found in soil, vegetables, human feces, and water. It has also been found in *human body lice* that were on homeless people living in France.

You will find Acinetobacter to be part of the skin flora of humans like the skin and mucous membranes, toe webs, groin, and axillae.

This organism is spreading rapidly and emerging with a widespread resistance to the newer antibiotics. This bacterium can become resistant at such a fast pace that it is quicker to do so than any other gram-negative bacteria.

They have a biofilm that helps them survive well in just about any situation.

Here we are back to the carbapenems as the treatment doctors lean on if the bacteria show any kind of susceptibility to it. Some programs favor imipenem as the potent antibiotic as compared with meropenem for treating a multi-drug resistant Acinetobacter infection.

Drug-Resistant Campylobacter

Sure, some of the organisms being discussed you will probably remark that you have never heard of in the news headlines. You probably have, or it was buried in the back of some magazine or newspaper but did not look like an article that interested you at the time and felt it was just a group of doctors blowing their pipe.

Campylobacter is something you NEED to be worrying about. How often have you heard someone in the summer say after being off work for a few days that they had a round of the stomach flu? More than likely it was no stomach "flu." In fact, they had a form of food poisoning and did not realize it.

Campy is one of the most common causes of gastroenteritis by bacteria and one of the most common bacteria that incites Guillain-Barre

Syndrome. You will also see Irritable Bowel Syndrome follow this infection.

Campy's favorite host is usually avian, but there can be other animal reservoirs. If you could see this bacteria under the microscope, you would see a something shaped like a comma, and it looks pink (gram-negative).

Don't get me wrong; it sits right by Salmonella and Shigella as another enteric pathogen.

The diarrhea is severe and can be grossly bloody. The abdominal pain can be so severe that many doctors will mistake it for appendicitis. You will most of the time see that the patient is better within a week, but some cases can keep relapsing for several weeks.

There is also a reactive arthritis that seems to happen in about 1 out of every 100 cases. It seems to occur about four weeks after the infection and usually affects the small joints of the hands, knees, wrists, and ankles.

Campy has become resistant to our sulfa drugs and is becoming more resistant to the fluoroquinolones in most areas of the world, so we are losing our traditional drugs of therapy. Right now, it seems that Macrolides are the drugs to be working the best but Campy coli is becoming more resistant, especially in China and other parts of Asia.

There is a worry for people traveling to underdeveloped countries. Even with the risk, prophylactic medications are not recommended for the travelers. Travelers must be advised to practice precautions such as only drinking bottled water. Eat only peeled or cooked fruits or vegetables (I would insist on only cooked because if the outside of the fruit were contaminated while peeling the fruit, the bacteria would be cut to the inside flesh of the fruit). Avoid any raw food coming from animals.

If you run into a Campy infection that has become life-threatening such as a blood-borne infection of Campy that is causing complications systemically, it would be considered reasonable to treat the patient with a carbapenem plus an aminoglycoside while waiting for culture reports to return.

Fluconazole-Resistant Candida

How many times have you known someone with a case of Candida? Especially a female friend. How many times have you had a male friend with a case of fungal infection in the groin area? Alternatively, how many times have you known someone who had a fungal infection under their toenails?

They are basically all the same in that they are a fungus. Fungus all have rods growing in every direction that spurts buds from them that then spurt more rods known in the science world as "hyphae" from that and it keeps growing until it looks like a big spider web and the worst part is that it causes severe itching of your flesh. For toenails, it turns them extremely hard, turns yellow and to release themselves from the nail bed itself and sometimes the toenail will fall off completely.

We have run straight into a brick wall for antifungal drugs that can save lives when the candida gets into the bloodstream. It is called antifungal resistance.

It seems to have been identified that Candida is now the most common reason of hospital-acquired bloodstream infections in the U.S. This one fungus can cause a patient to be in the hospital three to thirteen days longer and as much as $6,000 to $29,000 more in costs in healthcare monies.

It is one of the last organisms you would expect to be getting into someone's bloodstream and killing patients; but unfortunately, it is doing just that. It is quite sad watching the patient die as you stand by with nothing that will work to kill this organism.

What is of grave concern is that Candida is not only becoming resistant to the _first-line_ but the _second-line_ of antifungal meds that are being used.

However, you say surely there are other IV antifungals to fall back on; and you are right. What we see though, is that those medicines are very expensive to the patient and can be highly toxic to the patient that is already extremely sick, so the medicine given to them could kill them quicker than the infection.

Patients that do have drug-resistant candidiasis seem to have much poorer outcomes than those patients who have candidiasis that can be treated with the standard antifungal medications.

Just like Candida, Aspergillus (another fungus) is associated with a high mortality rate. Some of the studies on Aspergillus has identified that it may be driven by farmers using agricultural azoles (it protects their crops from fungus).

A patient on antibiotics for other reasons are at extreme compromise for developing Candidiasis as the antibiotics kill out the other normal flora in the colon leaving only the yeast to survive.

A farmer who had been cleaning out his grain bin came down with a terrible sinus infection. He could not get over it. He went to the doctor, but the antibiotics did not work on the infection. What the doctor's found was the infection, was that it was a fungal infection that had infected the meninges of his brain.

Antivirals were given IV to no avail. Nothing was working. His wife and each of his children was required to sign a statement that would release the hospital, the drug company, the pharmacy and all the healthcare professionals from liability from conducting this experimental procedure.

Then they started the procedure with the experimental drug by drilling a hole in the top of the patient's skull and dripping the drug straight down into the patient's brain. It did do the job it was intended for; it killed out the fungus growing in the man's brain. However, there was a downside. He was left with a brain of no more than that of a 12-year-old child until he died.

We become very desperate at times to keep our loved ones alive at significant costs with the outcomes. It seems we sometimes feel that the kill or cure method is at least a chance to have our loved one with us. When we do get our loved one back; sometimes we regret the decision we have made as we never get the loved one "we knew before" back. We get their physical body back, but never again see and enjoy the person we once knew before the experimental procedure.

Another potential reason for some of this resistance to candida is the use of over the counter antifungals bought so conveniently at all retail stores. It should be available to the consumer, but at the same time, maybe the ingredients should be changed every two or three years so that the yeasts and fungus we encounter every day do not become too accustomed to what we have and become resistant to what we utilize in our arsenal.

Extended Spectrum Enterobacteriaceae (ESBL)

ESBL is a bacterium that is quickly making headlines. It is a gram-negative or a gram-positive bacterium that has the potential to "create" its own enzyme (who said bacteria was not smart), and the enzyme is known as beta-lactamaze (an enzyme that can break down antibiotics) we primarily use to fight infections. The capability can be found in the cell of the bacteria in both the plasmids and the chromosomes. By breaking down the antibiotics, it takes away more of our agents with which to fight infections.

Two prime examples of ESBL producers are Klebsiella pneumoniae and Enterobacteriaceae E. coli; common bacteria that are usually the reasons for bacteraemia and urinary tract infections. Other ESBLS that have been reported are Serratia, Salmonella,

Pseudomonas, Proteus, and Enterobacter.

There are several reasons that someone might be at risk for contracting an ESBL and it does not mean you have to be in the hospital.

Here are a few:

- If you are living in a communal type living arrangement
- If you must wear an indwelling catheter
- If you must be tube fed, on dialysis, had an organ transplant, neutropenic
- If you have had to be in an ICU for a long time
- If you have had to be on antibiotics for an extended period

ESBL bacteria usually live in our lower colon of people who are infected. The most common way to transmit this organism is by unwashed hands.

Currently, we are looking at 30-50% of E. coli are resistance to amoxicillin and ampicillin due to beta-lactamase.

One summer while eating at a local restaurant an iced tea was ordered. As this person put the glass up to their mouth, it smelled like a sewer, and they could not stand to even think about taking a drink of it. It smelled so terrible they were unable to eat the meal that had been brought to them.

The tea was taken in a "to go" cup to the state lab before going back to work to have it cultured. It came back as E. coli! It, in fact, had feces in it of some type. It was not known how this large restaurant container of 'serve yourself' tea had become contaminated with feces, but it had. It was very contaminated as it grew out multiple colonies with a small loop.

It could have been contaminated on purpose by a disgruntled employee; an employee could have gone to the bathroom, defecated, not washed their hands after wiping, and come back and made the tea and had their hands down on the inside of the container carrying it back out to the drink section of the restaurant.

It does not matter how it was contaminated. It was disgusting, and this person has not been back to that restaurant for over ten years now.

If you want to understand why bacteria have been able to survive since the beginning of time think about it this way. Plasmids are the rings of extrachromosomal DNA on the bacteria itself, and it can be exchanged between different types, species of bacteria by conjugating, connecting, mating, joining up if you will. It can pass on to the other species it has been "conjugating" with its resistance genes.

As of this writing, the ESBLs are still susceptible to Cephamycins and Carbapenems. For how long, we do not know.

There was a 12-year-old girl admitted to the hospital with a high fever and pain in the right lower quadrant that would make you think appendicitis. She was given a 3rd generation cephalosporin for about four days. Her c-reactive protein was high, her white count was high, and her abdominal ultrasound showed a large abscess behind her cecum. Because of all the findings, she underwent surgery that same day. The pathological findings were gangrenous appendicitis, and it was positive for ESBL-producing E. coli. The only antibiotic that would work on it was carbapenem. The 12-year-old was in the hospital for 23 days before being released.

If you think like me, you are wondering how in the world did that bacteria get to be in an abscess behind her appendix? If you were to question any doctor, they would look at you and only shrug their shoulders, and they would not know either. Bacteria is a mystery of life.

    We do know the clinical implications are that treatments can still fail. ESBLs have come to be known as the ***Grim Reaper***. We know that there is a massive list of antibiotics that will NOT work on these organisms.

Vancomycin-Resistant Enterococcus (VRE)

This ugly bug has been around for quite some time. Since at least before 1992 one can say for sure. I fought this organism multiple times while serving as an infection control practitioner.

There was a well-known businessman who had a hernia that he kept putting off having surgery to correct. Then one day, the bowel at the sight of a hernia ruptures, spewing bowel out into his abdominal cavity. They rush him to surgery and operate to repair the damage and to try their best to clean his abdominal cavity out of the feces that had poured out into the abdomen. Multiple antibiotics are used on him. He develops a terrible infection despite all the antibiotics that have been pushed into his veins.

The doctors are at a loss as to what they can do for this patient. However, the Doctor of Pharmacy has an idea. There is a new drug just out on the market at the time called Zyvox that they might try. They could purchase this in IV formula to use for this patient. It was ordered. At the time Zyvox was new, and the price was astronomical for the IV formula. Today, the price of 28 tablets is $2,493.

The Zyvox, for which at that time there was no generic, was shipped in overnight and at 2:00 p.m. the next afternoon the IV was started. The patient responded quickly to the drug and improved daily until he could go home. You must remember that taking Zyvox has its risks. It is also, oddly enough, an MAO inhibitor and it has some not so good side effects and drug interactions. You must observe your diet carefully while on Zyvox as it can cause many interactions with typical foods, you would not expect.

When you observe this organism under the microscope, you will see what looks like a purple chain of pearls. It does not look dangerous, but dangerous they are; you can be assured of that fact.

VRE usually likes to live in the bowel and is resistant to so many antibiotics and even Vancomycin (considered the drug of last resort). VRE can cause urinary tract infections, sepsis (in the bloodstream), wound infections, meningitis, heart infections, pneumonia, and abscesses.

The two species mainly seen of enterococcus are Enterococcus faecium and Enterococcus faecalis which can both be vancomycin resistant.

If you have a Vancomycin-resistant enterococcus growing "conjugating" near or with a Methicillin-Resistant Staphylococcus Aureus, it can pass its plasmid properties to the MRSA and make the MRSA also resistant to the drug Vancomycin. NOT GOOD for the patient.

As it stands, about 30% of all the enterococcal infections we see are caused by VRE – Vancomycin-Resistant strains of enterococcus.

A person can carry VRE around in their body without it causing them any problems and not even know they are carrying it in their body. Most of the time they will be colonized in their bowel. If for some reason, the VRE numbers start to increase, they can enter the bloodstream, cause pneumonia, infect a heart valve, or an abdominal abscess.

Specific risk factors make one more susceptible to contracting VRE. Some of them are hospitalizations, IV lines, urinary catheters, undergoing gastrointestinal surgery, a compromised immune system for some reason, kidney failure, chronic disease such as being a diabetic, and cancer.

If you grow out VRE from anywhere and it cannot be treated by Vancomycin effectively, your state or territory lab and the CDC or, WHO should be contacted for further advice. An infectious disease doctor should be consulted as they may know some successful combinations of antibiotics to utilize.

Currently, to treat VRE, there is teicoplanin (not available in the U.S.), quinupristin-dalfopristin, telavancin, oritavancin, tigecycline, daptomycin, and linezolid.

If the VRE is in an abscess, it is crucial that the abscess is drained for the antibiotics to be successful. If your IV line is infected, they need to remove the line if possible since this is your source of infection. The same goes for urinary catheters.

Bottom line, VRE is not your friend either.

Multidrug-Resistant Pseudomonas aeruginosa

Do you remember Science Fairs when you were in school? Did you ever experiment culturing your mouth and then culturing your dog's mouth to show that your dog's mouth had fewer bacteria in it than yours did?

Did you ever see anything on your culture plate that looked kind of green and if you touched it with a loop or a toothpick it was gooey and stringy? Well, that was probably Pseudomonas aeruginosa. It just looks nasty and gooey growing on a petri plate. Pretty much like it does growing in your body.

Do not ever give it a chance to grow in your body. It likes a lot of warm moist places. It likes your bladder, your kidneys, your lungs, open wounds, fresh surgical wounds, and surgical site openings. It is considered an opportunistic pathogen. It is highly adaptable to many environments and seems to become comfortable where ever it lands.

    A female patient comes to the Emergency Room with the calf of her leg extremely swollen, inflamed and a large hole in the center that has turned black. The ER doctor asks her what has happened to her leg? She replies that she is not for sure, but thought she might have gotten a spider bite. He asks her why she thinks that and she goes on to explain that while she is cleaning out a closet, she felt a stinging sensation on the back of her leg and when she glanced around there is a large brown recluse spider on her leg. The doctor continues his questioning by asking her why she did not come in sooner with her leg. She replied that she had been putting ointment on it and was hoping it would get better.

    The cultures grow out the dreaded multi-drug resistant Pseudomonas aeruginosa. What now? The patient is taken to surgery multiple times to debride the calf of the woman's leg. It seems that it will never end and that they cut so much of the calf of the leg you can see the bone where the muscle of her calf once resided. Combination therapies are used along with multiple surgeries and a very lengthy hospital stay and then rehab so she can learn to walk with that leg again as most of that calf muscle is missing she finally gets to go home.

Pseudomonas is quite clever in being able to acquire its resistance. It can do so by the intrinsic resistance in which there is less penetration of that outside membrane of the bacteria, the discharge system of the organism that will actively pump the antibiotics right out of the cell of bacteria, and produce enzymes that will inactivate antibiotics.

There are about seven different combination therapies recommended to use MDR Pseudomonas aeruginosa again. This pathogen is scary and not just because of its high resistance but because of its uncanny ability to adapt. We MUST prevent the evolutionary pressure that can lead to emerging highly resistant clones.

Drug-Resistant Non-Typhoidal Salmonella

Your patient's family brings in their father who is 80 and says he has mental status changes in the last four hours. He has just seen his oncologist three hours from home and passed his oncology appointment with flying colors. On the drive back home, he sits quietly in the back seat which is not like him. Getting close to the town where the local hospital is located he says he needs to get out of the car.

You stop the car, and he gets out and just wanders around talking incoherently. Somehow you get him back in the car and head toward the Emergency Room. Something terrible has happened, and your first thought is that maybe he has had a stroke. You feel of him, and now he is burning up with a high fever! What has happened in the last four hours? You are stricken with fear and panic.

You get into the emergency room and explain to them that he has had severe mental status changes on his way back from his St. Louis oncology appointment. They rush him on back to a trauma bay and begin checking him. He asks immediately for what you think he is trying to say is a bathroom.

You assist him as he is still talking mumbo jumbo that no one can understand as he can barely hold his head up by now. He begins having horrible watery diarrhea and is so very ill, and his fever is 103.5 degrees. What has happened to your father?

You and your daughter call your mother and tell her what has happened, and you are in the emergency room trying to explain to them how quickly this series of events have taken place.

You speak with the doctor and tell him that this dropped out of the blue and you had no idea what has happened. He briefly mentions that he thinks it is no big deal and can probably be sent home.

Your hair stands on end as you again state to the doctor in a loud voice that everyone in the ER can hear; that this 80-year-old man has had severe mental status changes. He has 103.5 degrees of fever, and in case he cannot smell that putrid smell emanating from his room he needs to step into the trauma bay and take a whiff.

You tell the doctor, still in a very loud voice, informing him that he will not be sending your father home; he will be finding out what is wrong with this little man who is so ill and so precious to your family.

The doctor finally opens the doors to the trauma bay and goes in to see the patient. The most terrible smell finally hits the doctor and it spills out into the hallway. The doctor comes back out, orders admit and two pages of tests. He starts spraying air deodorizer throughout the entire ER. He **finally** gets your point.

Things start happening.

Blood draws are collected, x-rays are taken, and cultures are made of the stool specimens that are happening every 15 minutes. He is now losing blood quickly through every bowel movement. You keep wondering what has happened to this little man?

He is hooked up to fluids. His labs come back, and he is losing blood so quickly they are typing and cross-matching to start giving him blood. They continue giving him blood and fluids. He does not want to eat or drink. He says his stomach hurts so badly and severe pains are shooting through it. You keep asking yourself what has happened?

Two days later you finally have an answer. The cultures show he has Salmonella non -typhoidal. Antibiotics are started, there is no choice. His body cannot fight this bacteria on its own. He has not had chemotherapy for over ten years, but his Chronic Lymphatic Leukemia is starting to rear its ugly head again with a white count of 85,000 and almost 95% lymphocytes.

But, where did he contract this Salmonella strain? You keep thinking and trying to figure out where this has happened and how. Since you are such germaphobes at home, you knew it would have been impossible but still investigate possibilities of it happening there.

Finally, when your Dad is starting to make some sense and can think again, you ask him some questions. He admitted he had been having some diarrhea for a few days, but it was only two or three times a day. He even remembered when it started. That took us back to when and where and if he had eaten out at some restaurant lately, something he hardly ever did because of the germophobic family.

He remembered eating a grilled chicken breast sandwich and remembered what day he had eaten this sandwich. It all figured out. More than likely, someone had cooked the chicken breast but had used the same platter that the uncooked chicken had lain on to put the cooked breast back on before making the sandwich and it must have been covered in non-typhoidal salmonella. Alternatively, the chicken breast had not been cooked through and through as it should have been, and the organisms got into his gut that direction.

Had this not been caught when it was, and a few hours later, there could have been no coming back due to his health condition. The salmonella was already in his bloodstream. He was headed to sepsis.

It has now been four years, and he still has not eaten any chicken or turkey since that time. So, how do you feel about eating chicken at a restaurant now? This little man took almost three weeks regaining his strength.

Had this been a drug-resistant non-typhoid Salmonella I am not sure he would have survived this episode.

Infections from Salmonella can cause some severe complications if it gets into the bones, the central nervous system, internal organs or the bloodstream.

You can figure that most patients with cases of Salmonella will recover within five to seven days and not have any treatment whatsoever. However, if there is severe dehydration from diarrhea or severe bleeding with diarrhea, IV fluids and blood will probably be necessary.

Antibiotics are usually reserved for the severe cases that are high risk for complications.

We have about nine percent of the non-typhoidal Salmonella that is resistant to drugs and becoming more resistant to more drugs daily. One strain of Salmonella, a serotype called "I" was 46% multi-drug resistant four years ago. Three years prior it had been 18%; therefore, it had more than doubled in three years. These numbers are quite frightening for our future. This serotype is linked to consuming **beef** or **pork**, and that includes meat bought at live animal markets.

A female patient decided to buy some Holy Water from an advertisement seen in a magazine. She received the Holy Water from somewhere overseas and instead of using it for sprinkling; she drank it because she had been having pains in her stomach.

The female patient came into the hospital unresponsive. Blood cultures grew out the drug-resistant Salmonella. The family brought in the bottle of Holy Water, and it was cultured as well. It too grew out the same strain of Salmonella. Apparently, the Salmonella had been able to enter her bloodstream through an ulcer in her stomach that she had not known she had; but if she had seen a physician she could have been appropriately diagnosed.

Once the root of the problem was identified a combination of antibiotics were given, and the patient slowly recovered.

We are facing each year, infections from foodborne organisms that are antibiotic resistant causing about 440,000 illnesses in the U.S. alone.

Many people do not realize that those cute little green turtles that people keep for pets and some reptiles carry salmonella. It is not just found in poultry, fowl of all kinds, and many other sources that you would not even think about being contaminated by Salmonella. Sometimes some species are found in cat and dog diarrhea specimens that can be transferred on to humans and even though the human will more than likely recover; they may shed the bacteria for months later; meaning they can pass it on to someone else.

Drug-Resistant Shigella

Here we have another very common food poisoning closely related to Salmonella.

Foreign travel is becoming riskier. Moreover, it does not mean "just don't drink the water risky."

It has been identified that people traveling internationally are bringing in this multidrug-resistant stomach bug to the U.S. and freely giving it to those who have not traveled.

Shigella sonnei that was resistant to ciprofloxacin caused 243 people to get sick in 32 states in less than a year. Cipro was at one time the first choice in treating shigellosis.

Shigellosis can spread faster than wildfire in daycare facilities, bisexual and gay men, and homeless people. Just in the United States, we see resistance to Shigella by sulfa and ampicillin. We have found that doctors here in the U.S. have been prescribing to people who travel abroad, Cipro just "in case" they get diarrhea while traveling. It could be affecting the resistance to Cipro by Shigella.

If you are traveling to other countries, try to protect yourselves by eating only the very hot foods (not spicy hot, but steaming off the stove hot) and drink liquids only from untampered sealed bottles.

In the United States alone Shigella causes about 500,000 cases of diarrhea each year. It can spread rapidly from one person to the next.

If you are traveling abroad take bismuth subsalicylate to keep from getting travelers' diarrhea and if you do get diarrhea try treating it with the bismuth subsalicylate or loperamide. Use antibiotics as a last resort. That is easy for the scientists and doctors to say if they are not the ones having diarrhea every fifteen minutes.

It seems that once you have had a Shigella infection, you will probably not catch it again for several years. However, you can still become infected by other strains of Shigella. There is at the time of this writing, research to develop a live oral vaccine to keep you from getting Shigella. However, will the Shigella remake itself like the flu and the vaccine not work?

Drug-Resistant Streptococcus pneumoniae

You come home from working in the field and cannot find your wife anywhere in the house. You keep calling her name, yet she still does not answer. You know she has not been feeling good lately and has had a severe sinus infection, but she is stubborn and will not go to the doctor.

You go through the house again and notice in one bedroom that the bed covers do not look quite right where she had made the bed, and you look between the bed and the wall, and there she lay unconscious with blood running from one ear.

Frightened, you pick her up and rush her to the nearest hospital. There they find she has had such a severe sinus infection that she had also developed an ear infection that had ruptured her tympanic membrane in her ear and the multidrug-resistant strep pneumoniae had entered to the meninges of her brain, and she had developed meningitis from the drug-resistant strep pneumoniae. She never regained consciousness after you found her and died three days later.

This Multi Drug-resistant Streptococcus pneumoniae carries a high mortality rate. It does not respect age, creed, or color. It causes all kinds of severe infections that are life-threatening like septicemia, meningitis, and pneumonia. It ALONE can be held responsible for the deaths of over one million people a year around the world.

Every year just in the United States Strep pneumoniae will be responsible for about 3,000 cases of meningitis; 50,000 cases of bloodstream infections; and 7,000,000 ear infections.

This ugly bug is spread by droplets that come out of our mouths when we talk, laugh, sneeze, sing, or cough. It can also be passed to each other by direct contact.

There are some people who are considered carriers. In their case, people may carry the strep pneumoniae in the back of their throat, and it never causes a problem for them, but they can pass it on to others.

Drug-Resistant Strep Pneumoniae are no more virulent than any other pneumococcal infection, but they can become seriously ill very quickly.

You could be vaccinated against this disease, but most people will not do so, because most insurance companies will not cover this expensive vaccine, but they will cover the 15-variety pneumonia vaccine.

Methicillin-Resistant Staphylococcus Aureus (MRSA)

MRSA has been plaguing Infection Control Practitioners and Physicians for years now, and it is not getting any better. It seems to be the norm in nursing homes. If you do not have MRSA, you are considered odd.

When MRSA and VRE are growing in the same tissue alongside each other, they are capable of exchanging plasmid properties with each other. The Vancomycin Resistant Enterococci can make the Methicillin Resistant Staph Aureus also resistant to Vancomycin leaving an MRSA that cannot even be treated with Vancomycin, the usual drug of choice.

Our athletes seem to be having problems with this ugly bug as well. It seems they are culturing it from their wrestling mats and multiple wrestlers on the wrestling teams are coming up with MRSA boils on various parts of their bodies.

Some cities are encouraging their residents to use the so-called clean water that has been filtered from the city sewage plant to water their lawns with during the summer to save on the city's water supply. What they also found was that the incidence rates of MRSA skyrocketed in their towns and when tested the water coming from the filtered city sewage plant was rampant with MRSA.

You may not believe it, but they have identified "Fido," your favorite household pet as being the number one culprit of carrying MRSA in your home.

There are so many cases of babies and toddlers not yet potty trained that come through the ER and pediatrician's offices with boils on their bottoms underneath their diapers that it is appalling. When the boils are lanced and drained and then cultured, they almost always culture out MRSA. What is causing this? Where is this coming from? We have not been able to identify the culprit at this point.

At present, about 33% of the population is carrying staph in their nose, and that is usually if they have no illness. You will have about two in every one hundred that will carry MRSA in their nose.

MRSA can be picked up in the hospital or the community. They call it CA-MRSA for community-acquired or HA-MRSA for hospital-acquired.

However, MRSA is not just resistant to methicillin. It has become resistant to many other antibiotics as well. Plasmid properties have been shared by other bacteria and made it resistant to other antibiotics.

MRSA has been the culprit for causing necrotizing fasciitis (means "causing tissue death"). This is what you may hear on the news as flesh-eating bacteria. If you have never seen this phenomenon, it is hard to believe what you see before your eyes. After you have seen it, it seeps into your dreams at night and comes back to haunt you years afterward.

When the flesh starts to be eaten by the bacteria, you can watch the flesh die and turn black sometimes faster than an inch an hour. It makes it hard for the physician to get ahead of the bacteria to cut off what he can to stop the movement of the bacteria in its eating frenzy. If it is not stopped, it will eat the patients entire body. It can be deadly before you know it.

Once necrotizing fasciitis gets inside your body, it infects your fascia, the connective tissues that encompass your muscles, fat, blood vessels, and nerves. At times, the bacteria will produce toxins that will also cause more tissue to die. It can cause the patient to have loss of limbs or die.

It is rare that anyone can contract necrotizing fasciitis from anyone. It seems to occur randomly. It can enter your skin only by a cut, a burn, insect bite, puncture wound, or a scrape. Never take anything for granted.

People who contract a flesh-eating bacterium will usually observe soreness or pain at the scratch site, kind of like a "pulled muscle." Your skin may start to feel warm and then purplish and red areas of swelling will spread rapidly. There are some people who will develop blisters, black spots, and ulcers on their skin. As the flesh-eating bacteria progresses, you will start to have chills, vomiting, fever, and fatigue. If ANY of this happens to you, seek medical attention IMMEDIATELY!

A gentleman had come in for abdominal surgery. He was recovering well and had been discharged home with his staples in place five days after surgery. He could walk around in his yard but be careful and just rest. He was doing amazing after his surgery. Three days after going home he reappeared back in the emergency room. His abdomen around the surgical incision site was black, and it looked like the black was moving as the doctors examined him!

There was no guessing to what organism this was eating away at him right before their eyes. From somewhere, after he had gone home, he had contracted a flesh-eating bacterium. He immediately was taken back for emergency surgery to try and get ahead of the bacteria. His flesh had to be cut back to the sides of his ribs. His internal organs left open but covered by some solid mesh until they could do skin grafts for this gentleman.

If he had not rushed back to the hospital when he did, by the next day he would not have had to come to the hospital. I know this is hard to believe if you are not a medical person. It is true. It is frightening. This is our wake-up call.

Sometimes MRSA can start on the skin and just look red or like a rash. It may have a pimple or a boil, and they may be filled with pus. From there it can start weeping pus and draining fluid. Alternatively, it could come up as an abscess as I discussed above about the babies' diapers.

MRSA is very infectious and so easy to contract by touching someone who has it or by touching a surface in a room where they have been. It can live on a surface for days.

We find that people who get MRSA sepsis or pneumonia usually have a death rate of about 20%.

Once you get MRSA, you usually are colonized for quite some time, and MRSA can live for days and weeks on hard surfaces. You can carry it on your clothes and your shoes and then track it into your house. Anyone crawling or laying on your floor can pick it up from there.

During a statistics and data summation of all the babies and toddlers coming through our emergency room with MRSA boils under their diapers there was a discussion with one of our pediatricians. We asked her what her recommendation was for children to prevent the boils.

She informed us that when her children were bathed at home, a small amount of bleach was added to their bath water in the event there were harmful pathogens being carried on their skin.

You will find some that say, "Kids need to get used to dirt and germs, that is the problem now." They are uneducated and do not understand what is happening. The children are already subjected to normal bacteria every day, and that is what they should be exposed to; however, they should not be subjected to multidrug-resistant pathogens such as MRSA that could become life-threatening in the small child if left untreated.

Drug-Resistant Tuberculosis

Most people think that tuberculosis is a thing of the past. Let me tell you my friend; it is far from that. Tuberculosis is alive and well and waiting or its next host to live inside their lungs. This drug-resistant strain leaves us with fewer options for treatments, and this can cause the increase in the risk of death.

Tuberculosis is usually in the lungs, but it can spread out to other organs. The frightening part is that it is spread when someone who has TB laughs, talks, coughs, or sneezes. The TB germs can float in the air for hours. People who breathe in this air can then become infected with TB.

When we discuss multi-drug-resistant tuberculosis, we are referring to a form of TB that is caused by a mycobacterium that is resistant to at least two of the first-line drugs used to fight tuberculosis and this is isoniazid and rifampin. Scarier still is that we have some forms of tuberculosis that are now resistant to the second-line drugs!

It is understandable how this is hard to believe, but about one in four are infected with tuberculosis worldwide. Infection with TB is different when it becomes active and starts causing symptoms such as coughing; blood tinged sputum, shortness of breath, night sweats, and weight loss.

We are finding that the multi-drug resistant TB is being found responsible now for 75% of the cases of tuberculosis today.

There were 480,000 new cases of multi-drug resistant TB cases in 2015 and 250,000 deaths. When you are looking world-wide most of the MDR-TB cases are found in Southern Africa,

China, India, South America, and what was known as the former Soviet Union.

Many cases of MDR-TB are due to people who do not finish their full course of medication therapy.

It has been witnessed that in the last ten years there have been some TB strains in India, Iran, South Africa, and Italy that are resistant to all the first and the second line drugs for TB. These have been classified as TOTALLY DRUG-RESISTANT TUBERCULOSIS.

Some people cannot take the tuberculosis drugs because they are so hard on the liver. It is especially true for the elderly patient.

Prisons have extreme difficulty with MDR-TB in their prison populations and no wonder they are all housed in such close quarters day in and day out breathing the same air.

Many patients do not want to take the medications for the six months or more that is required to rid them of this disease, making more and worse drug resistance. It is a lose, lose situation. Health departments must provide directly observed therapy to those patients to assure they are compliant with their medication rituals.

Before government cutbacks, there were tuberculosis "sanitariums" ran by each state where only patients with TB went to be treated and cared for until they were cured. The TB facilities were a good program because the patients were watched as they took their meds each day, so they never missed a dose and they were there until cured. Cure rates were better and less chance of developing resistance to drugs.

Chapter 5: Where Do We Go from Here?

What are we going to do? We worry about our children going to school because there might be one of their classmates come to school with a gun and kill them that day.

We worry about North Korea lopping a nuclear warhead over on anyone he chooses and frying everyone in its path, as well as the ground for miles around.

We worry about the next tsunami that MIGHT happen if we live near the ocean or if the volcano in Yellowstone National Park is finally going to erupt and, if it does, what exactly will happen when it does.

We worry about if California's big quake will ever happen and part of California will ever fall into the ocean taking with it millions of people.

However, we seem to never worry about organisms that can kill swiftly and painfully, and we cannot start to see them with the naked eye.

We think when we go to the doctor we still expect an instant fix and never dream that we have contracted a multi-drug resistant organism.

A nurse friend was taking B12 injections every week at home, so her husband was assisting with the injections. She noticed one morning there was an extensive and angry raised red area around the injection site about five inches in diameter. She made an appointment and went to her primary care physician who immediately had her admitted to the hospital.

She died three days later, leaving a husband and three-year-old daughter. She had developed MRSA at the injection site because the area had not been cleaned properly before the injection. It quickly went to her bloodstream, and she became septic shutting down her organ systems one by one until she was pronounced dead. She was 32 years old.

At risk of being a dooms-dayer; we could be looking at a terrible future on our horizon. A future that will rip one of the most valuable tools for a doctor right out of his hands. The very thing we held up as the "Miracle" will become our downfall: antibiotics.

We may soon be seeing a time when a simple cut on your thumb could cause you to be left fighting for your life.

We will see a time when a mole removal or appendectomy could become a death sentence.

Organ transplants and cancer treatments will kill you. Childbirth, once again, could become deadly in a woman's lifetime.

You may think this book has read like science fiction, however the stories have been real.

If there would be new drugs that keep coming, we would not have to worry, but there have not been any "new class" of antibiotics developed since the 80s; which in and of itself is frightening to those who realize what is happening.

In London, the patients used to be placed in beds outside to breathe in fresh air as the cure for tuberculosis. They either lived, or they died. Since we are running out of drugs for tuberculosis, this is what it will look like for our future.

We are facing an antibiotic "apocalypse". It is coming and faster than you ever thought it could come...

How will you be ready?

Conclusion

I am going to say that those of you reading this book may think that this was a dooms-day prediction and do not want to hear what is said. I respect that and that is fine. You do not have to believe what is written herein. You can choose to learn more by browsing the Center for Disease Controls website and the World Health Organization, and they will have the same messages for you.

You were given case scenarios, so that you would have examples of how quickly and swiftly death can come from some of the Super Bug infections.

All of the multidrug-resistant organisms have not been discussed here. Only the most frequent have been spoken about. There are a lot more. It is what is happening now.

In our household all fruits and vegetables, even watermelons, cantaloupes, and bananas that will be eaten raw are all bleached in a 1:100 bleach solution for ten minutes and then rinsed with clean tap water or bottled water and left to drain. When dry they are then placed in new, clean bags with paper towels to keep them fresh and free from all pathogens that could harm.

When and if you mix up Clorox at your home, please bear in mind that it will only retain kill properties for 24 hours. After that time, it will turn back to a salt and no longer have any kill potential. You must mix fresh every 24 hours.

Cantaloupes are famous for their rough surface to have Listeria monocytogenes on the outside. When you cut through them, the pathogens can then pass to the fruit inside, and you can ingest the Listeria. Listeria can cause miscarriages in pregnant women.

Never order ice water with a slice of lemon. You have no idea as to how this lemon has been handled and if it has even been cleaned before slicing and placed in your glass of water or if it might have feces on it from the worker picking the fruit.

We can't deny it. Antibiotic resistance has changed everything we cherished from the "miracle".

How interesting it is that something so small, something that can only be seen with a microscope, can outsmart mankind. It has gained power over us, for which, unfortunately, we have no arsenal to fight.

**Welcome to the
Post Antibiotic Era.**

www.ingramcontent.com/pod-product-compliance
Lightning Source LLC
Chambersburg PA
CBHW071058240526
45471CB00016B/2103